I0412560

understanding
DIABETES AND GLYCEMIC INDEX
SELECTED TIPS - 75 PAGES!

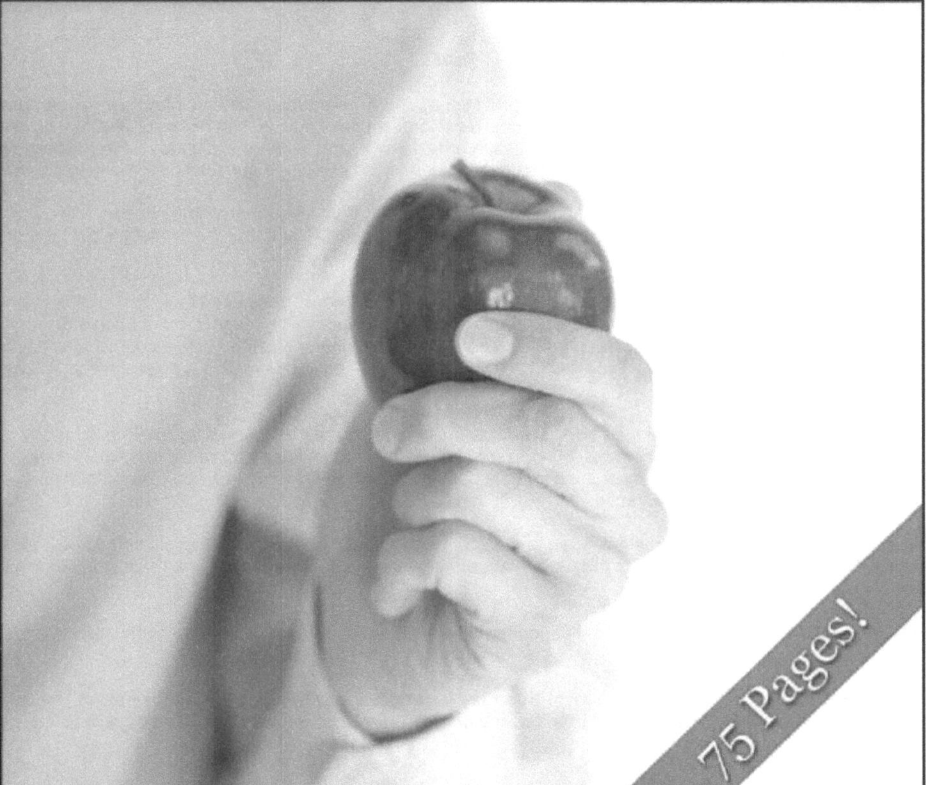

Understanding Diabetes And Glycemic Index

75 Pages!

Brought to you by Wings of Success

Understanding Diabetes and Glycemic Index

DISCLAIMER AND TERMS OF USE AGREEMENT:

(Please Read This Before Using This Report)

This information is not presented by a medical practitioner and is for educational and informational purposes only. The content is not intended to be a substitute for professional medical advice, diagnosis, or treatment. Always seek the advice of your physician or other qualified health provider with any questions you may have regarding a medical condition. Never disregard professional medical advice or delay in seeking it because of something you have read.

Since natural and/or dietary supplements are not FDA approved, they must be accompanied by a two-part disclaimer on the product label: that the statement has not been evaluated by FDA and that the product is not intended to "diagnose, treat, cure or prevent any disease.

The author and publisher of this course and the accompanying materials have used their best efforts in preparing this course. The author and publisher make no representation or warranties with respect to the accuracy, applicability, fitness, or completeness of the contents of this course. The information contained in this course is strictly for educational purposes. Therefore, if you wish to apply ideas contained in this course, you are taking full responsibility for your actions.

The author and publisher disclaim any warranties (express or implied), merchantability, or fitness for any particular purpose. The author and publisher shall in no event be held liable to any party for any direct, indirect, punitive, special, incidental or other consequential damages arising directly or indirectly from any use of this material, which is provided "as is", and without warranties.

As always, the advice of a competent legal, tax, accounting, medical or other professional should be sought. The author and publisher do not warrant the performance, effectiveness or applicability of any sites listed or linked to in this course.

All links are for information purposes only and are not warranted for content, accuracy or any other implied or explicit purpose.

This report is © Copyrighted. No part of this may be copied, or changed in any format, or used in any way other than what is outlined within this course under any circumstances. Violators would be prosecuted severely.

Contents

Nutrition And The Glycemic Index

Eating healthy means knowing the nutritional value of the foods we eat. Although once that only meant vitamins and minerals, we now have a new area: the glycemic index of carbohydrates. What this does is give us an indication of how the sugar is being used in the body, and which carbohydrates have higher sugar content and should be restricted. Certain carbohydrates turn to sugar more so than others, and thus create the potential for high blood sugar. Some of these products are easy to identify such as cakes, candies, and other sweets, but it also includes other products such as potatoes, refined white flour, white rice, and even white bread.

Learning to eat carbohydrates that have a lower glycemic index is one step toward having a more nutritionally balanced diet. In addition, these products are more likely to keep your energy level to be at its height of performance, thus preventing mid-morning or mid-afternoon sluggishness that often results from skipping breakfast or consuming foods that are too rich in quick sugars. The carbohydrates that have a lower glycemic index create slow burning energy that keeps a person going longer in addition to maintaining that full feeling that prevents overeating.

For the person who has had trouble with weight in the past, the switch to low glycemic index carbohydrates will be a welcome change. Often people eat either because they need energy or because they feel they are hungry, but the way these carbohydrates work in the body will help with both of those issues and thus a person can eat less, maintain a high energy level, and feel full longer between meals. It will take a little time to become used to the transition, but once you learn new eating habits, you will not want to return to your old way of eating.

The Glycemic Index: Preventing Diabetes Through Diet

For those who are prone to diabetes, a change in diet is the best way to prevent or slow its onset. That means the consumption of carbohydrates that have a low glycemic index so that less sugar is being stored in the bloodstream. This, of course, will not help those who already have diabetes, though it will certainly help keep the blood sugar level under reasonable control – that does not mean you will be able to stop taking your medication, as that is something that is contingent upon your personal case history and your doctor's recommendations.

Aside from those who have diabetes in their families, another risk factor is a woman who develops diabetes during pregnancy. Even if no one in your family has ever had the disease, if you develop it during pregnancy, chances are higher than normal that you will develop it later in life. The transition to a healthier way of eating and a switch to low glycemic index carbohydrates can either prevent or delay the onset. After all, you will be gaining more energy and losing sugar from your bloodstream, so it is reasonable to assume that diabetes will be delayed and even prevented.

If you already have diabetes and are on medication for it, the switch to low glycemic index carbohydrates may alleviate some of your symptoms and keep your blood sugar level under better control. This is especially helpful for those who have found it difficult to keep it under control with medication and diet – perhaps you are eating foods that are actually turning to sugar in the bloodstream, which is what happens with carbohydrates that have a high glycemic index. Reducing the amount of high glycemic index carbohydrates will definitely make a difference in your blood sugar level and help alleviate some of the symptoms that are connected to your diabetes.

The Glycemic Index: Lifestyle Changes

In order to remain healthy in our later years, lifestyle changes are needed that include changing the way we eat. Even if you think you are eating healthy foods, look at what you are eating in the way or carbohydrates. If you are eating white bread, white flour, white rice, potatoes, and cereals that are not in the oat, bran, or barley group, you are eating carbohydrates that have a high glycemic index. That doesn't mean you are going to be able to eliminate all of the carbohydrates that have a high glycemic index, but the goal is to reduce them so that less sugar is going into the blood stream and more is being utilized and turned into energy. The body needs the energy for your to feel rested after a good night's sleep, but you want to consume the slow burning energy rather than the quick energy that is derived from sugar products such as candy, cakes, and other sweets.

Diet and exercise are important to good health, but you want to make sure that you are eating foods that are nutritionally sound. Don't go by things you were taught in school unless you are very young because things that were taught about nutrition ten, fifteen, and twenty years ago have now been changed. While many of us were taught that slow burning carbohydrates included potatoes, white bread, and unsweetened cereals, we are now finding that only a portion of that is correct information. As years go by, science finds out different information about the foods we eat, so it's important to make certain that you have the most current information before you make any lifestyle changes. For this, the Internet is the most reliable source of information since web pages are changed on a regular basis as opposed to a book that you may pick up in the library or bookstore.

The Glycemic Index: Is It Worth The Effort?

When you consider the difficulty that is involved in making changes in the way you eat, the first thing people tend to wonder is whether it's really worth it. When you go on a diet and have to give up or reduce your intake of certain foods, you ask yourself that question, and it has to be an answer with which you can live. If you are overweight and want to lose weight, of course, changing the way you eat will be worth it. The same holds true for switching your eating habits to low glycemic index carbohydrates. Certainly, the body is going to go into shock from the change, but in the future, it will be worth it as you find that you have more energy, your mind functions better, and your health is better.

Changes in eating are never easy, especially not if you have been eating the same way for many years, and if that involves a great deal of unhealthy eating. Lifestyle changes are never easy, but if it's for the benefit of your health, present or future, it's worthwhile to make the effort. Remember, even if you have no health issues at the present time that require you to switch to low glycemic index carbohydrates, the benefits on your future health as you age are enormous. In addition, the earlier you begin eating differently, the easier it is for both you and your family to adjust to the changes. Making a change after twenty years of high cholesterol eating is much more difficult than making the same change after five or ten years. Don't wait until you have a health issue such as the onset of diabetes to make the change; do it now before your doctor forces you to do it because of your health.

The Glycemic Index: It Seems More Difficult Than It Is

Making a transition to a healthier eating style is not as difficult as it seems at first; unless you are one of these that have his mind made up that you don't like wheat bread or whole grain cereal. If you make the changes with a positive attitude, you will achieve far greater success than fighting the transition or doing it "because the doctor made me do it." You have to do it because you know it's the best thing for your health and because you want to do it. Unfortunately, that sometimes means a health scare that shakes you into reality, thus the reason that so many people fail when they try to change the way they eat.

Making a lifestyle change is all in the perception of it. If a person is really adamant they do not want to do it, then they are going to make it more difficult than it needs to be. For instance, switching to whole wheat bread is a simple transition on a low glycemic index carbohydrate diet, but if a person insists that they "hate" that kind of bread, the transition is going to be more difficult than if they accepted it as part of a regiment of healthy eating. Quite often people fail at diets and other lifestyle changes because they want to be contradictory and insist that they don't see the point in making the changes or "what is the difference if it's white bread or wheat bread" kind of attitudes. It's much like the pregnant woman who is told she can only have one soda per day and insists, "What is one more?" The more difficult you attempt to make the task, the more difficult it will become.

Making lifestyle changes for the benefit of your health can be easy if you allow them to be. You are in charge of the transition to the lifestyle changes, and if you make it difficult, it will be. If, however, you accept that it is for the good of your health, the transition will go smoothly and effortlessly.

Depression And Diabetes

Many people who are diagnosed with diabetes are overwhelmed with an onslaught of new information, medications, doctor visits and a feeling of helplessness. Diabetes can be frightening, particularly for anyone who is not familiar with the disease. We read about complications and insulin and medication and feel hopeless.

Many diabetics experience a period of denial when first diagnosed with diabetes. They refuse to believe there is anything wrong with them. While they remain in denial, the condition worsens. This can often lead to depression. Depression and diabetes often go hand in hand. According to the American Diabetes Association, people with diabetes have a greater risk for developing depression than other individuals.

The stress of management of diabetes can take a toll on an individual. There are new medications to take, blood sugar must be monitored frequently and a record kept for your doctor. There are frequent doctor visits and there may be several different medication combinations needed before your blood sugar is kept under control.

On top of that, people who have diabetes are often faced with sudden lifestyle changes. Foods that they once enjoyed are now taboo. An exercise regime is often recommended, which can be good for depression, but people with depression often have little energy to begin an exercise regime. As the depression continues, people often lose interest in monitoring their blood sugar levels and may even skip their medication.

Symptoms of depression include a loss of pleasure in every day activities you used to enjoy as well as a change in appetite. You may have trouble concentrating and have trouble sleeping. Or you may even sleep too much. Many people suffer from depression, but for a diabetic, it can be life threatening. Depression and diabetes is a dangerous combination.

People who are diagnosed with diabetes can empower themselves by learning as much about the disease as possible from the beginning. This can alleviate the feeling of helplessness that often accompanies the diagnoses. Ask your physician questions. Do research. Find out how you can help manage you disease.

Understanding Diabetes and Glycemic Index

If you feel you are suffering from some of the signs of depression, ask your doctor to recommend a therapist who is familiar in dealing with people with chronic illness. Therapy can be crucial for a diabetic patient who feels isolated because of all of the extra work involved in treating their illness. Do not be afraid to discuss your illness with family and friends. Diabetes is a nothing to be ashamed of, it is a disease that affects millions of people.

If at all possible, join a support group for others who also have diabetes. Here you can not only find kindred spirits who are experiencing some of the same fears as yourself, but you can also learn new information.

Any time someone is diagnosed with an illness puts them at risk for depression. Their world has changed and no longer feels safe. Worse of all, they feel out of control. If you are diagnosed with diabetes, take back the control and learn how to manage your disease. By empowering yourself, you will not only be able to effectively manage your diabetes, you will eliminate the depression.

Diabetic Diet

Vigilance regarding your diet can not only help you control your diabetes, but can also eliminate the need for insulin. Many people with Type II diabetes are often prescribed tablets or pills in an attempt to control their condition prior to having to use insulin. By following a proper diabetic diet, someone diagnosed with Type II diabetes, which has reached epidemic proportions throughout the United States, can either prolong the need for insulin or continue to treat their condition with more convenient medications.

People with diabetes have a difficult time breaking down carbohydrates in their system. Carbohydrates are a large group of foods that are necessary for a balanced diet. While many people assume diabetics must avoid sugar, this is just one example of carbohydrates. In addition to foods rich in white sugar, carbohydrates include white bread, pasta, rice, potatoes, some vegetables and fruits as well as anything rich with white flour. Carbohydrates are a complex group of foods and different groups cause different effects to the blood stream. While diabetics have a difficult time breaking down any carbohydrates in their blood stream, those with the highest Glycemic Index rating take the longest to break down in the blood stream and cause the most harm.

By following a diet with limited amounts of carbohydrates, being aware of the Glycemic Index and learning which carbohydrates are the most harmful to a diabetic diet, someone with this potentially life threatening condition can keep this disease at bay. If you have recently been diagnosed with Type II diabetes and have been given medication by your doctor as well as diet suggestions, follow the doctor's instructions. Diabetics tend to be in denial more than any other group of patients and remain the most non compliant. By following a good diabetic diet and taking your prescribed medication, you can live a full and normal life span.

A diabetic diet should include limits on carbohydrates and increases in protein. Sugars should be eliminated as well as white flour. Pasta and rice are also rich in carbohydrates. One way someone can follow a good diabetic diet is to follow some of the low carb diets that were popular some years back. Many of these diets either eliminated or limited carbohydrates. There are also many different diabetic cookbooks for those with this condition that can help a person live a happier, healthier life.

Understanding Diabetes and Glycemic Index

It is unfortunate that so many people are continuing to be diagnosed with diabetes. The good news is that there is plenty of information out on the market with regard to cookbooks and even on the internet regarding how a diabetic diet can help someone with this disease. Diabetes takes a toll on the human body after a certain period of time. By following a good diabetic diet, one can reduce the toll of the disease and live a longer and more fruitful life.

Those with diabetes should become aware of the gylcemic index, follow a diabetic diet, see their doctor regularly, monitor their blood sugar and take their medications as prescribed in order to avoid complications that can arise from this disease.

Gestational Diabetes

According to the American Diabetes Association, about four percent of pregnant women develop gestational diabetes. Gestational diabetes is a condition in which a woman who has never had diabetes develops high blood glucose levels while pregnant, usually within the later term of the pregnancy. It is estimated that there are about 135,000 cases of gestational diabetes every year in the United States.

In most cases, women who develop gestational diabetes will not develop Type II diabetes. This is a condition affected by the pregnancy and the inability of the mother to use the insulin naturally developed in her body. It is caused by hormones triggered by the pregnancy and causes the mother to become insulin resistant. Gradually, the mother develops high blood glucose levels, referred to as hyperglycemia.

Normally, a woman with gestational diabetes will be treated for the condition while pregnant. While there are no birth defects associated with this sort of illness as there are with women who have had diabetes prior to being pregnant, there is generally not a large cause for alarm for the child. However, if the condition is left untreated, it can hurt the baby. Because the mother is not getting rid of her excessive blood glucose, the child is getting more than his or her share of energy and fat. This often results in macrosomia. Macrosomia is simply the clinical name for a fat baby.

While some people think a fat baby is the sign of a healthy baby, a child born too fat may have a problem fitting through the birth canal. This can cause shoulder damage and may require a cesarean section birth,. In addition, babies who are born obese can develop breathing problems and, if they remain obese, may themselves develop Type II diabetes.

Fortunately, there is treatment for gestational diabetes. Insulin injections are usually given to the mother to keep the blood glucose levels intact. A woman who is planning on becoming pregnant, however, can avoid the complication of developing gestational diabetes prior to becoming pregnant. Some of the ways a woman can do this is to lose weight if she is already overweight prior to becoming pregnant, develop a healthy exercise routine and follow certain food guidelines. The Glycemic Index is an ideal tool for a woman who is thinking about

Understanding Diabetes and Glycemic Index

becoming pregnant to use to determine which foods to avoid. The Glycemic Index was developed for diabetics to categorize carbohydrates for those with diabetes.

When you become pregnant, follow the advice from your doctor regarding diet and exercise as well as any carbohydrate diets. Prior to becoming pregnant, discuss any concerns you have regarding weight or diabetes with your physician as he or she can probably give you some advice on how to avoid this pregnancy complication.

Even if you are diagnosed with gestational diabetes, chances are that you will not develop Type II diabetes, neither will your baby and both of you will be just fine. Gestational diabetes is not a reason to panic. There is plenty of care available for women with this condition. Just be sure to follow any instructions given to you by your doctor.

Glycemic Index

The Glycemic Index is a concept developed in the University of Toronto in 1981. The purpose of the Glycemic Index is to measure the effect carbohydrates have on blood glucose levels. The Glycemic Index is imperative for anyone who needs to monitor their glucose level due to diabetes or hyperglycemia. With diabetes reaching epidemic levels in the United States, the development of the Glycemic Index could not have come at a better time. Each year, more people are diagnosed with this potentially life threatening disease that can cause many serious complications. It is important for anyone with this condition to familiarize themselves with the Glycemic Index so they can empower themselves and learn which foods should be avoided.

Carbohydrates are a diverse group of foods and all have different ways of breaking down in the system. People with diabetes have a difficult time breaking down certain foods, particularly those high in carbohydrates, in their system. Digestion is slow and sugars and starches are absorbed into the blood stream, causing an excess in blood glucose. Diabetics are often warned to limit their carbohydrate intake because it takes such a long time for most carbohydrates to digest. However, this is easier said than done and it is difficult, if not impossible, for many diabetics to eliminate carbohydrates from their diet. This is one of the reasons many diabetics are non-compliant in their treatment. Because diabetes does not often cause serious complications at onset, many patients refuse to take their medicine and continue eating foods that are high in sugar and starch.

The Glycemic Index is very helpful because it rates different carbohydrates based upon their effect on the different levels of blood glucose. Those foods that digest rapidly cause the less harm to the system and have a low glycemic index. The carbohydrates that take a longer time to digest have a higher rate as they cause more harm to the blood glucose level.

The Glycemic Index ranges from one to one hundred. A low food in the glycemic index has a rating of below 55. These include fruits, vegetables, whole grains and some pastas. Foods that fall between the 56 to 69 range are considered "medium" in the Glycemic Index. They include candy bars, croissants and some rices.

Surprisingly, although a candy bar scores in the medium classification of the glycemic index, it is not as harmful as those carbohydrates that score in the high glycemic index range. These

Understanding Diabetes and Glycemic Index

include corn flakes, white rice, white bread and baked potato. In other words, it is easier for a diabetic to digest a candy bar than a baked potato.

Knowledge of the glycemic index is imperative for anyone who has diabetes or who has been diagnosed as borderline diabetic. To be able to understand which foods have the most impact on blood glucose levels is crucial for anyone fighting this potentially life-threatening condition.

If you or a loved one suffers from diabetes, become familiar with the Glycemic Index so that you learn about the different categories of carbohydrates and which groups should be avoided. There are many substitutes for carbohydrates that rate high in the Glycemic Index and are available at most grocery stores. While diabetes is currently without a cure, there are many different ways that people with this disease can life long, productive lives.

High Glycemic Foods

In 1981, Dr. David Jenkins of the University of Toronto came up with a ranking system for carbohydrates based upon how long it takes them to break down into the system. Some carbohydrates break down very slowly and those release glucose gradually into the bloodstream and have a low glycemic index. For people who are diabetes, particularly those who are insulin dependent, a low glycemic index is preferable. These foods allow the insulin or medication to respond better to the blood glucose and allows for the sugars to break down more naturally.

Other foods are rated high on the Glycemic Index. These foods currently have high ratings and raise the blood glucose level quickly. High glycemic foods can be beneficial for people who are recovering from high exertion or those suffering from hypoglycemia. People with Type I or Type II Diabetes should avoid high glycemic foods as they can play havoc with the insulin or medication they are taking.

Some examples of foods that considered high glycemic foods include corn flakes, white rices such as jasmine rice, white breads and baked potatoes. People who have diabetes, either Type I or Type II, should avoid these foods as much as possible.

Other foods that are high glycemic foods include those with large amounts of white refined sugar or white flour. One thing a doctor will tell a patient on how to avoid high glycemic foods is to avoid anything white. This includes white bread, pasta made with white flour and even cakes or sweets made with refined white sugar or white flour.

High glycemic foods tend to take a long time to digest in the system of a diabetic. The glucose, or sugar, stays in the blood because the system of a diabetic is unable to process the refine sugars and flours. The glucose stays in the blood and in the urine causing the diabetic to frequently urinate, experience thirst and hunger more than the average person and sweat profusely.

After a while, this takes its toll on the system of a diabetic. The kidneys begin to hurt because they are not functioning properly. This is one symptom that diabetics often present with when seeking a physician. They also get blood in their urine and, in the worst case scenario, they

Understanding Diabetes and Glycemic Index

faint or enter into an episode of semi-consciousness, confusion which can even lead to a diabetic coma. In some instances, a diabetic coma can prove fatal.

People who have Type I and Type II diabetes should be very mindful of which foods have a high glycemic index and avoid these foods in their diet. With proper diet, medication or insulin and monitoring of blood sugars, diabetics can lead a normal lifespan.

Diabetes is not a death sentence at all. It is simply a condition that many people possess that does not allow their body to break down sugars and starches through their system so that they digest normally. Diabetes is harmful to an individual who does not follow the advice of their physician, does not consume a proper diet and does not monitor their blood glucose levels. People who adhere to the medical guidelines concerning diabetes have just as much of a chance of living a normal life as anyone else.

How To Prevent Diabetes

In many instances, diabetes is an inherited disorder. People who have first degree relatives with this disease are more prone to developing this disease than people with no genetic disposition. People who have a first degree relative with diabetes can avoid contacting the illness by having themselves tested by their physician. The physician can do a series of blood tests that will determine whether or not the patient is pre disposed to this condition. If a person has a pre diabetic condition, there are many things they can do to avoid getting this disease.

However, Type II Diabetes has become nearly an epidemic in this country. Many in the medical community believe that one of the reasons many people acquire this potentially life threatening condition is from obesity. The diabetes epidemic has mirrored the obesity epidemic currently overtaking the United States as well as other countries. People consume foods that are high in carbohydrates and sugars and low in nutrients at an alarming rate. We often think of diabetics as being people with a sweet tooth who crave sugar. This is not the case. More often, a person who is obese has more of a chance of getting diabetes than a person who maintains his or her weight.

One way how to prevent diabetes is by managing your weight. Although there is little you can do about having a genetic disposition to the disease, there are ways you can prevent becoming one of the millions of Americans who develop diabetes each year.

When seeking how to prevent diabetes, the first thing a person can do is watch your weight. Studies indicate that people who are overweight are more prone to developing diabetes. How to prevent diabetes. Rule number one is manage your weight. One way to manage your weight is to stay way from foods laden with saturated fats, and sugars. Stay away from fast food, which is usually high in fats, carbohydrates and sugars. Most fast food offer little in the way of nutrition but are high in fat and carbohydrates.

Another way how to prevent diabetes is to exercise. Exercising regularly improves blood sugar control. Because active muscles dispel glucose from blood quicker than non-exercised muscles, regular exercise can do wonders in staving off or preventing diabetes. In addition, regular exercise also helps to maintain stable weight, another factor in preventing obesity.

Understanding Diabetes and Glycemic Index

Again, the misconception that people contract diabetes through excessive consumption of sugars is inaccurate. It is not only sugar that contributes to the disease. While it is good to eliminate the use of excessive sugar in your diet, carbohydrates are also contributory to the onset of diabetes. One way on how to prevent diabetes is becoming aware of the Glycemic Index. The Glycemic Index was developed in 1981 and rates which carbohydrates are more difficult to eliminate glucose from the blood.

When asking yourself how to prevent diabetes, focus your attention on your weight, exercise and diet. In many cases, simple lifestyle changes can prevent someone from getting this potentially life threatening disease.

Insulin To Treat Diabetes

When someone has Type I diabetes, which used to be referred to as Juvenile Diabetes, insulin is the natural treatment. In this case, a person does not produce any insulin and insulin must be injected in order for the patient to survive. Just as there are many different types of oral medications to treat Type II diabetes, there are also many different options when it comes to insulin to treat diabetes.

Years ago, insulin was derived from animals and injected by a needle. Patients often needed multiple insulin injections throughout the day. There were problems with the insulin derived from beef and pork and many patients developed a resistance to the insulin after a period of time. In 1977, modern technology in the treatment of diabetes took a giant leap as human insulin was cloned. Today, insulin to treat diabetes is human insulin and is much more effective than insulin used in the past.

There are many different types of insulin on the market today and, as is the case with oral medications, it may take several different insulin types in order to find the correct balance that will insure good glucose levels. Some insulin, such as Humalog, is very short acting and peaks within an hour after injection. Other insulin, such as Ultra Lente, is very long acting and peaks in 18 hours.

There are three characteristics to insulin. Onset is the time it takes for the drug to reach the bloodstream and begin lowering the glucose. The peak time is the time when the drug is at the maximum strength and the duration is how long the drug continues to work in reducing the blood glucose level.

Each patient has different needs when it comes to insulin and for this reason, there are many different types of the drug. Cost is also a consideration in many cases as the insulin must be injected every day and, in certain instances, many people have to inject the insulin several times a day.

Another benefit of modern technology in managing people with diabetes through the use of insulin is the insulin pump. This is much more effective than injections as it is a catheter that remains under the skin and separates the insulin into three different types of insulin. Basal

Understanding Diabetes and Glycemic Index

insulin is injected continuously. Bolus doses are given to cover any carbohydrates consumed in a meal. You can also have correction doses or supplemental doses. This is especially effective if your blood sugars are high prior to eating.

The use of the insulin pump is much more effective than using injections as it controls your insulin and blood glucose levels on a continuous basis. It is relatively easy to use and most people with Type I diabetes are using insulin pumps.

Not only people with Type I diabetes use insulin. Those with Type II diabetes who have been unable to control their blood sugars through diet and medication are often prescribed insulin. Because the insulin pump is so effective at retaining control of the blood glucose level, many people with Type II diabetes have also opted to use the insulin pump.

Medical science is continuing to search for a cure for diabetes which has reached epidemic proportions in some areas. Until a cure is found, however, there are many ways to treat this disease. When someone gets a diagnoses of diabetes, they often panic and are overwhelmed at all of the information. If you or a loved one is diagnosed with diabetes, become empowered by learning all you can about treating the illness, learning about different medications and making sure that you comply with orders given by your physician. Patients with diabetes who are compliant and learn about their disease stand the best chance of living a long and productive live, despite having diabetes.

Kidney Disease And Diabetes

Not everyone who has diabetes gets kidney disease. This is yet another popular misconception about the illness. While uncontrolled glycemia can cause kidney disease, diabetics who maintain their proper blood glucose levels can avoid kidney disease.

Diabetics who get kidney disease acquire this life threatening condition because they are unable to dispose of the waste products of sugars and starches through their systems. These foods remain in their system and do not break down and eliminate, as they do in others without the disease. The sugars and starches stay in the system and cause the blood sugars to rise to high levels that can be dangerous. Not only that, it makes it difficult for proteins to pass through the system.

Eventually, when a person has uncontrolled diabetes and does not maintain their proper blood glucose levels, the elimination process through the kidneys ceases to function effectively. The kidneys have to work harder and harder to eliminate the waste products and the proteins are blocked. The kidneys filter too much blood and begin to leak. Protein is lost through the kidneys and from the body. Towards the end, waste products begin to build up into the blood.

This is the basics of kidney disease. Kidney disease is acquired in many ways. In diabetics, it is acquired because the kidneys worked too hard to filter out the sugars and starches and were unable to remove waste products from the blood. Eventually, like any organ that is overworked, they shut down. When the kidneys shut down, a person is often put on dialysis, in which a machine functions as the kidneys. In some cases, a person with kidney disease can opt for a transplant, however this is not often available to persons with diabetes.

A person cannot live without their kidneys. Therefore, it is imperative that a person with diabetes understands how their kidneys function and what they can do to help these vital organs function efficiently. A diabetic does not have to contact kidney disease at all. A diabetic can avoid most complications of the disease by simply following the orders of their physician and maintaining a healthy lifestyle.

Many diabetics are non compliant patients. Non complaint patients are those who do not do what the doctor instructs them to do. They do not follow the diet as recommended in the

Understanding Diabetes and Glycemic Index

Glycemic Index. This chart was developed to inform people with diabetes of which foods to avoid. Those foods that are high in the glycemic index take the longest to break down and do the most damage to the kidneys, who try their best to eliminate the waste. The Glycemic Index was developed in 1981 and is a potential lifesaver for anyone with this disease as it clearly states which foods to avoid.

Other methods of non compliance include not monitoring their blood sugar. A diabetic is often prescribed a blood monitor that he or she must use several times a day to check their blood glucose levels. In addition, the levels are recorded and should be presented to the physician during their scheduled visit. Many diabetics do not comply with this integral part of their treatment.

Insulin or medication is usually prescribed for diabetics who sometimes refuse to take these lifesaving medications. The insulin or medication enables the foods to break down and assists the kidneys in eliminating waste. There is no reason not to take these medications and there are many different programs available for those who cannot afford these medications.

Exercise and weight control are crucial to maintaining a healthy lifestyle not only for diabetics, but for the general population. Yet many people simply refuse to follow these essential guidelines.

Diabetes is not necessarily a precursor to kidney disease. Kidney disease and diabetes are two different diseases. One does not always lead to the other.

Link Between Diabetes, Heart Attacks And Strokes

Diabetes is a disease in which the body either lacks insulin or does not produce enough insulin to break ingested glucose into cells. As a result, the glucose remain in the blood and damage blood vessels. A high content of glucose in the blood is called hyperglycemia and is often a precursor to heart attack and stroke. People who have diabetes have twice as much of a chance of having a heart attack and stroke as those without this condition.

In addition to diabetes itself being a risk factor for heart attack and stroke, there are other risk factors that people with diabetes should be aware of to reduce their risk factor for heart attack and stroke. This includes central obesity. Studies by the American Heart Association have indicated that while obesity in itself is a risk for a heart attack, carrying excess weight around the waist increases your risk of heart attack. This is believed to be due to the fact that abdominal fat increases bad cholesterol more than fat on other areas of the body.

Speaking of cholesterol, those with diabetes should carefully monitor their cholesterol carefully. Because the blood vessels are already weakened by the excessive glucose in the blood level, people with diabetes have to be especially careful about their cholesterol levels as their arteries can become blocked easier than those without diabetes. Monitoring cholesterol is important for everyone, but imperative for those with diabetes.

Hypertension is also a dangerous condition for those with diabetes and can lead to heart attack or stroke. Damaged blood vessels having to work harder to pump blood from your heart throughout your body can cause heart damage, stroke, and even eye problems.

Clearly, those who have diabetes must not only carefully monitor the disease, but he complications that can rise from diabetes. While it is important for everyone to check their blood pressure, cholesterol and maintain an ideal weight, it is even more important for someone who has diabetes.

In order to reduce the risk of heart attack and stroke for people with diabetes, it is important, first of all, to manage the disease. By eating proper foods that are recommended for people who have this condition, exercising and taking your medication, you can maintain a good glucose level in your blood that will reduce your risk of heart attack and stroke. By monitoring

Understanding Diabetes and Glycemic Index

your cholesterol and blood pressure and seeing your physician on a regular basis, you can stop a potential problem before it begins.

By empowering yourself to learn all you can about managing diabetes and complying with the instructions of your physician, you can live an active and long life with diabetes. Knowledge and facing the situation is the key. Those who refuse to follow advice, who prefer to eat whatever they feel like, not exercise and pretend that the disease does not exist put themselves at the most risk.

Type II diabetes is reaching epidemic proportions in the United States. It does not have to be a killer. People who follow instructions, learn about the disease and comply with their physician have an excellent chance at reducing their risk of acquiring any of the complications associated with this disease. Despite the link between diabetes, heart attack and stroke, those who maintain their health can avoid these conditions.

Medications That Treat Diabetes

Currently, there are many different medications that treat diabetes. Most people who are diagnosed with Type II diabetes are given medication instead of insulin. In most cases, a combination of drugs are used. These drugs work with the body to increase insulin production and make it easier for the body to eliminate glucose.

Sulfonylureas are one of the most popular drugs used to treat diabetes. There are several different types of this drug on the market, the most popular being Glucotrol. These drugs work by increasing the amount of insulin released from the pancreas. These drugs work well in lowering blood glucose levels but also run a risk of a person developing hypoglycemia. Hypoglycemia is when the blood sugar level is too low. Because of this potentially dangerous side effect, sulfonylureas are often given with other drugs, most notably Glucophage, or more commonly known as Metformin. This drug works well with Glucotrol as it reduces the amount of glucose in the liver while the Glucotrol increases the amount of insulin in the pancreas. Both medications must be taken prior to meals. Most people who are first diagnosed with Type II diabetes are given this combination of drugs which, when taken as directed, are effective at maintaining a healthy blood glucose level.

Another drug that is showing promise in working well with Metformin is Prandin. Prandin also lowers blood glucose levels but at a slower rate than Metformin and has shown good results in studies. Like Glucotrol, Prandin increases the amount of insulin in the body and can also cause hypoglycemia. It is very important for a patient with diabetes to work with their physician to get the right dosage of each medication and never double a dosage or cut one in half. Prandin cannot be used in women who are pregnant or nursing children.

Starlix is another drug that works similar to Prandin but does not require adjustments. The dosage remains constant and is also safe to use on those with kidney problems. Starlix is yet another promising drug being used to treat people with Type II Diabetes.

While most medications that treat diabetes increase insulin developed in the pancreas and decrease the glucose in the liver, newer medications are being marketed that decrease the absorption of carbohydrates in the intestines. Precose did remarkably well in trial studies in breaking down the carbohydrates in the system, making it easier to eliminate. However, this

medication has not done as well as the sulfonlureas, which are considered the best possible medications that treat diabetes at this time. However, for those who are allergic to sulfur, Precose is a good alternate.

Other new medications that are concentrating on controlling the glycemic control in the system include Symlin and Byetta. While these drugs have proven to be show promise, more testing is needed before they can replace traditional therapies.

A diagnosis of Type II diabetes may be frightening for an individual, but there are many different medications available that can keep this disease at bay. It is very important, however, for a patient to be totally complaint in order for these medications to work effectively. It may take increased dosages, lowered dosages or different combinations of medications in order to get the right balance that will help you maintain a healthy blood glucose level. This is why it is so important for an individual to carefully monitor their blood glucose level throughout the day and keep a record for the physician.

By working with your physician and reporting symptoms and results of blood glucose monitoring, you can empower yourself to keep your diabetes in check and avoid any complications that are associated with this disease.

Pre Diabetes

Type II Diabetes has become somewhat of an epidemic of late. More and more people are being diagnosed with this potentially life threatening condition. Type II Diabetes usually sets on later in life, although more younger people are being diagnosed every day with this disease.

According to the American Diabetes Association, approximately 54 million people in the United States have pre diabetes. Pre diabetes is a condition in which the blood glucose levels are higher than normal but not high enough to be considered Type II diabetes. Although pre diabetes is not a full fledged disease, it can also cause complications in the heart and blood circulation if left untreated.

The good news about pre diabetes is that with proper nutrition and the care of a physician, you can avoid being diagnosed with Type II diabetes. The condition can reverse itself, but it does take work on the part of the individual, as well as compliance with the orders directed by your physician.

Obesity is also an epidemic in the United States and many in the medical community believe that this is contributory to the corresponding diabetic epidemic. It is the general consensus of the medical community that obesity is a precursor to Type II diabetes. Therefore, those who have pre diabetes can stave off the disease by making some healthy life choices that will eliminate their need for medication or insulin in later years.

One way to reverse the effects of pre diabetes is to maintain a healthy weight. This can be easily accomplished through diet and exercise. For those who feel that it is too much trouble to manage their weight or complain that they do not have the time to exercise, they need to realize that the time they spend exercising now can eliminate their time spent on dialysis. While not all people with diabetes experience kidney failure, many do. And when the kidneys fail, these patients must spend many hours each week, hooked up to a machine that functions as their kidneys.

Those who complain that they do not want to watch their diet can be reminded that it is easier to watch their diet than to inject themselves with insulin or monitor their blood glucose levels several times a day. Those who feel that foods that are rich in carbohydrates are less

Understanding Diabetes and Glycemic Index

expensive than healthier alternatives can be reminded of the cost of medications and doctor visits for those who refuse to take control of their condition right away.

While some people are pre disposed to diabetes through genetic factors, others acquire this disease by eating too many bad carbohydrates, being inactive and not maintaining a healthy weight. If you have been told that you have pre diabetes, do not fret. You can reverse this condition. Begin an exercise regime, even if it only entails walking. Take a look at the Glycemic Index that explains which foods diabetics should avoid and follow these suggestions.

See your doctor about being put on a weight loss program and make certain that he or she continues to monitor your blood glucose levels. Pre diabetes does not have to turn into Type II diabetes. By developing a healthier lifestyle, you can reverse this condition and lead a longer, healthier life.

Symptoms Of Diabetes

Diabetes is a disease that is generally determined by the concentration of glucose in the blood. The amount of glucose in the blood is glycemia. The Glycemic Index indicates which carbohydrates have the highest levels of concentration of sugars and starches that make it so difficult for some diabetes to digest. Most diabetics have either Type I or Type II Diabetes. Generally, when a person is diagnosed with Type II diabetes, they are generally adults. Many people develop Type II Diabetes later in life after experiencing certain symptoms.

Diabetics have a difficult type processing certain foods, such as sugars and starches, into their digestive system. Certain signs of diabetes include frequent urination, increased thirst and desire for fluids and may also include an increased appetite. In many cases, a person with Type II diabetes feels generally unwell but cannot figure out what is wrong. Symptoms can mirror the flu or other illnesses. If you are experiencing frequent thirst, excessive urination and a substantially increased appetite, have yourself checked out for diabetes.

Fatigue is also a symptom of diabetes and Type I Diabetes may cause loss of weight, despite increased eating. The reason for the symptoms is because of the glucose concentration in the blood, also called glycemia. Because the glucose concentration is raised beyond the allowed threshold, glucose remains in the urine, causes more pressure and more frequent urination. When uncontrolled, diabetes can cause kidney edamage.

Some patients with Type I diabetes present with nausea, abdominal pain and an comatose state. Diabetic ketoacidosis is another term for a diabetic coma which can result when diabetes is undiagnosed or uncontrolled. A diabetic coma can result in death.

Most people with diabetes have too much sugar in their blood. There is another type of diabetes, however, called Hypoglycemia, in which the patient has a lower than normal amount of glucose in the blood. This can result in a variety of symptoms including fainting, feeling poorly, impairment of functioning and even coma.

If you have symptoms of diabetes, you should check your blood sugar level with your doctor. Although more definitive tests are needed to properly diagnose diabetes, high or low blood

Understanding Diabetes and Glycemic Index

sugar can be an indicator that you should see your doctor to determine the cause of the abnormal blood glucose.

Symptoms of diabetes can be frightening, but are easily controlled. If you feel that you have any of the above listed symptoms, do not be afraid to see your physician. Diabetes, although seemingly scary, is easily controlled. Physicians know more about diabetes now than ever before and there are many effective medications on the market to keep your disease under control.

If you have a family of history of diabetes, are overweight, or have not have your blood sugar tested recently, be aware of the symptoms of diabetes and have your physician test your blood the on your next visit. If you begin experiencing any of the symptoms of diabetes prior to your physician visit, do not be foolish - go to the ER and have yourself checked out.

The Effect Of The Glycemic Index On The Body

The Glycemic Index was discovered in 1981. It determines the rates of how different carbohydrates effect the body. The Glycemic Index is especially important to those who suffer from diabetes who need to watch their blood glucose. Diabetes have a difficult time breaking down glucose found in many carbohydrates and digesting them normally. This causes kidney and sometimes liver damage   The effect of the glycemic index on the body is that it allows people to know which carbohydrates are the ones that can cause the most damage and those that break down easily in the system. The effect of the glycemic index on the body is crucial to anyone who wants to monitor their blood glucose level.

For example, certain foods, such as vegetables and fruits, with the exception of the potato, can be good glycemic foods. They are low on the glycemic index and tend to take a long time to break down in the body, giving the system plenty of time to absorb the sugars and eliminate them without causing too much damage to the body. Other good glycemic foods include whole wheat pastas and certain types of rice. There are many excellent whole wheat pastas on the market today that make a wonderful substitute for traditional pastas that are made from white flour.

By being aware of the glycemic ratings, the effect of the Glycemic Index on the body can also assist a person who wants to avoid those carbohydrates that absorb quickly into the system and are the most difficult to digest. These include white breads, refined sugars, baked potatoes, rice, items made with white flour. By understanding he ratings of these carbohydrates, a diabetic can be educated to know the effect of the glycemic index on the body.

Years ago, people with diabetes would simply be told to avoid carbohydrates. It was not until 1981 when the medical community began rating different carbohydrates as to their impact on the system. It became apparent to medical researches that certain carbohydrates absorbed quickly into the system and others absorbed more naturally and were more desirable alternatives to the high-rated carbohydrates. By 1981, the medical community was discovering he effect of the glycemic index on the body not only pertaining to diabetics, but to others as well. The effect of the glycemic index on the body gave birth to some very popular low-carb diets such as The South Beach Diet and other diets that monitored carbohydrate ratings.

Understanding Diabetes and Glycemic Index

The effect of the glycemic index on the body can assist a person who is watching his or her carbohydrates, either due to diabetes or a diet, to determine which carbohydrates are more dangerous for their body than others. A person who has been diagnosed with diabetes should familiarize him or her self with the Glycemic Index as soon as possible.

Diabetes can be controlled by a healthy diet. By learning about the Glycemic Index, one can empower themselves to learn which foods should be avoided and which foods can be beneficial to their health. All individuals can benefit from the Glycemic Index, but this information is particularly invaluable to someone with diabetes.

Weight Control In Diabetes Management

It is imperative for a person with diabetes to manage their blood sugar and carbohydrate intake. This is the objective of diabetic management. Unlike people without the disease, diabetics do not process certain sugars and carbohydrates through their system, which increases the glucose level in their blood,. Glycemia is the term used for the measure of glucose in your blood. People who have diabetes have to measure the amount of glucose in their blood several times a day. Monitors are provided to people with diabetes by their physicians so that they can do this. There are many different monitors on the market today that make monitoring blood glucose levels easy and painless.

There are several reasons as to why certain people are prone to acquiring diabetes. Although there is a genetic link to the disease, weight also plays a significant role in diabetes. People who are considered obese have an increased chance of acquiring diabetes and poor weight management makes it difficult for them to control the disease.

People who are overweight can, in some cases, eliminate the condition by losing weight. If, for example, a significant gain in weight caused a person to acquire Type II Diabetes, a proper diet and elimination of the obesity can reverse the condition of the disease. Weight control in diabetes management is not only essential in treating the disease, but can also actually reverse this potentially life threatening condition. There have been many instances where those who have been obese and who have lost weight have also lost diabetes. This reversal effect, however, only works with those who contacted the disease by being overweight. Those who contact diabetes through a genetic disposition cannot reverse the condition.

Weight control in diabetes management can take many facets. From eating the correct foods and eliminated carbohydrates, particularly those that are high on the Glycemic Index, from your diet, you can not only lose weight, but manage the disease.

Exercise is crucial for everyone. It raises our energy level, keeps us active, improves our mental state, is instrumental in treating depression but is essential when managing diabetes. By exercising, a person with diabetes can not only better control the glucose in their blood as active muscles can better eliminate blood glucose than idle muscles, but exercise is an excellent way to implement weight control in diabetes management.

Understanding Diabetes and Glycemic Index

Weight management in diabetes is one of the more important aspects of treating this condition. Other ways in which someone can manage their diabetic condition is to take the proper medication as prescribed by your physician and be certain to monitor your blood glucose with a testing device. Many diabetics, especially when first diagnosed, are in denial. Diabetes are among some of the most non compliant patients treated by physicians, which can be dangerous to the patient and frustrating to the doctor. By following doctor's orders, eating the proper foods, taking prescribed medication, monitoring your blood sugar levels and watching your weight, you can stave off harmful complications of this disease. Weight control in diabetes management is one of the first methods in treating your condition,.

You Can Control Diabetes

Perhaps you, like many other Americans, have recently been diagnosed with diabetes. Diabetes can be a life threatening condition and can cause many different complications in individuals with this illness. If you or a loved one has recently been diagnosed with diabetes, be aware that you can control diabetes. By maintaining your weight, following the instructions of your doctor and taking your medication, as well as watching your diet, you can eliminate the complications that often arise in someone with this condition.

There are many ways you can control diabetes. Many people who are first diagnosed have a period of time where they are in denial. Although Type II diabetes has become somewhat of a national epidemic, many people refuse to believe that they could possibly have this disease. Perhaps they are not overweight or do not eat a lot of sweets. These are only two precursors to diabetes. Many people who are not overweight or who do not eat a lot of sugar have also been diagnosed with Type II diabetes. It strikes everyone. And there are also some indications that it can be an inherited disorder. If you have a first degree relative who has diabetes, there is a very good chance that you may inherit this disorder. You should bring this matter to the attention of your physician so he or she can do some simple blood tests to determine if you are at risk for diabetes.

You can control diabetes. If you are diagnosed with Type II diabetes, one of the first things you need to do is to get a blood sugar monitor so that you can keep a record of your blood sugar. Your doctor will want you to do this several times a day, particularly after you eat. You will also, most likely, be prescribed certain medications. You should take them as directed. You will also be given diet suggestions.

Many people who have Type II diabetes are non compliant. This means that they do not take their medicine, monitor their blood sugar and eat all the wrong things. You can control diabetes if you simply comply with your doctor's instructions.

One of the best things you can do to control diabetes is by being aware of the Glycemic Index that is given to certain carbohydrates. Those with Type II diabetes are warned to stay away from carbohydrates. Diabetics have a difficult time breaking down the sugars and starches and absorbing them into their system. Certain carbohydrates have higher blood glucose levels

Understanding Diabetes and Glycemic Index

which takes them longer break down. By being aware of which carbohydrates rank high in the glycemic index is just one way to monitor the glycerin, which is the amount of glucose in the blood. It is imperative for a diabetic to monitor their glycemia.

You can control diabetes if you take your prescribed medication, monitor your blood sugars, become aware of carbohydrates that are high in the gylcemic index and keep an eye on your glycemia, which is the concentration of glucose in the blood. By complying with medication, testing and diet, you can keep your diabetes under control.

Purpose Of The Glycemic Index

Carbohydrates react in different ways on the glucose levels in our blood. In spite of what many people think, not all carbohydrates affect the blood sugar level in the same way, and to avoid the potential for high blood sugar that can take a toll on our health, it's important to know which carbohydrates produce the lowest amount of sugar in the bloodstream.

Knowing the glycemic index of the foods you eat allows you to choose foods that have a lower glycemic index, meaning making choices between those carbohydrates that produce less sugar in the bloodstream. The purpose is multi-level because it allows you to maintain good help, keep your weight understand control, and prevent diabetes and heart disease. It's important for one to know the foods that are have a lower glycemic index in order to know which ones are healthier.

Quite possibly all of us were taught that complex carbohydrates were the slow-burning sugars, thus created the slow burning energy that kept us going through the day in comparison to sweets such as cakes and candies that gives us a quick lift but a quick burn out as well. In other words, we were taught that a slice of bread, pasta, or a potato were better for us than a candy bar, and although that still holds true to a degree, it is not totally factual. Starches are no longer considered complex carbohydrates as we were taught, but are still in the category of simple carbohydrates that turn into sugar as they are digested. On the other hand, whole grains such as brown rice, sweet potatoes, whole wheat flour, whole grain cereals, and non-white breads do not have the same effect and thus have a lower glycemic index than their white counterparts.

The importance of the glycemic index cannot be stressed enough, especially with all we know today about diabetes and heart disease. In the past, we consumed various food products and never knew the harmful effects, but to continue to do so with modern knowledge is courting disaster. Now that we have the knowledge, it's important to take the time to research the foods we eat, especially carbohydrates, and choose those with the lowest glycemic indexes. Being more careful what we eat will make our lives longer, healthier, and more meaningful.

The Importance Of Knowing The Glycemic Index

How important is it to know the glycemic index of the carbohydrates that you consume? That depends on how closely you want to monitor those you eat. It is, of course, possible to simply follow the lead of others and switch to certain foods that you know have a lower glycemic index, but if you want to know what that figure is, it helps you retain more knowledge about the foods that you are eating. Once we know what we are eating and what is in the foods we consume, it makes it an easier transition to eating something that is healthy.

For those who are not used to eating carbohydrates based on their glycemic index, this will be a new experience, and with that comes the need to know just how it is going to affect your body. You want to know what you are putting into your body and why these foods are healthier than the ones you have been eating. As consumers, it's important for us to know just what we are buying and the ingredients in those products in order to know that we are not consuming something that is not good for us to consume. The same holds true for a low glycemic index carbohydrate diet – why would you not want to know the glycemic index of the foods you are eating? If you are going to take the time to make the switch, you may as well take the time to learn all of the facts about what you are eating as well as the information about the products that you used to eat.

Before you make the switch to a low glycemic diet, make certain that you know just where you want to be and then do the research. Information is available that will give you both the glycemic index and the glycemic load of many different foods. Having a diet that is nutritionally well balanced and healthy means knowing the contents of the carbohydrates you consume and whether they fit into the glycemic index where you or your doctor wants them to be When you know this information, it is much easier to know just how much of a difference the change in foods is making on your body's energy level and overall well-being.

Benefits Of The Glycemic Index

While we used to think that starches were complex carbohydrates, we have since discovered that only whole grain starches can boast of being a complex product. Those include whole grain breads and cereals, brown rice, sweet potatoes (rather than white potatoes), and whole wheat pastas and noodles. Certainly, they are healthier than eating cakes, candies, and other sweets, but the body still turns them into sugars when they enter the bloodstream. They may have a lower glycemic index than the quick sugars, but nonetheless, their glycemic index is still too high to afford much in the way of healthy eating.

If one wants to be healthy, it's important to limit the amount of high glycemic index foods you consume because these types of foods push your body to extremes. This is especially true if your weight is above healthy limits and you lack exercise. If you do nothing more than switch to eating mostly low glycemic index carbohydrates that allow a gradual release of glucose into your blood stream, your energy levels will become balanced, and you will be less likely to become hungry in between meals.

Some other benefits that one can derive by eating carbohydrates with a lower glycemic index include:

- Ability to lose and control weight
- Increase in insulin sensitivity in the body
- Improvement in diabetes control
- Reduction in the risk of heart disease
- Reduction in cholesterol levels
- Better management of PCOS symptoms
- Reduction of hunger and ability of the body to stay full longer
- Increase in physical endurance
- Assistance in re-fueling carbohydrate stores after exercise

When one has trouble with weight that in itself can lead to diabetes, so it's important to be careful of foods that may add sugar to your bloodstream such as those with a high glycemic index. It's an overall benefit of good health as well, and if, in the process, you can prevent the onset of diabetes and heart disease, it is worth the effort. Adding some exercise to a diet rich in

Understanding Diabetes and Glycemic Index

low-GI carbohydrates will certainly provide a great deal of assistance when it comes to preventing diabetes and any of its related complications. Even if you have had it all of your life, watching your intake of high glycemic index carbohydrates will improve the body's ability to keep your blood sugar under control.

<u>Making The Switch To A Low Glycemic Index Diet</u>

It's a difficult transition switching from eating carbohydrates that are unhealthy to those that are healthier because of a low glycemic index. However difficult it may be, your health depends upon your consumption of a healthy diet that includes whole grain products and unbleached flour instead of the white products that you have been accustomed to using. It's not that difficult a decision to make, but it means a difference between being healthy and continuing a lifestyle that is or may be detrimental to your health.

Choosing a diet with a low glycemic index is not difficult and doesn't require a great deal of thought. You are not giving up foods, but you are eliminating carbohydrates that have a high glycemic index and replacing them with carbohydrates that have a low glycemic index. There is no need to count numbers of do any arithmetic in order to make sure that you are eating a healthy, low glycemic index diet. The easiest way to do that is by doing the following:

- Eat breakfast cereals that include oats, barley, and bran
- Eat breads that contain wholegrain, stone-ground flour, or sour dough
- Reduce the amount of potatoes you eat
- Eat plenty of fruits and vegetables
- Instead of white rice, use Basmati or Doongara rice

The initial switch is difficult because you will be eating differently that you have been accustomed all your life, but when you body begins to feel better, and you find that you have a higher energy level, you will see how much healthier a lifestyle that you have. Making any kind of change in your eating habits is difficult, whether it's a reduction in sugar, carbohydrates, or reducing the size of the portions you eat. When you are used to eating a certain way or certain foods, the transition period is very difficult.

If every one of us would grow up eating healthy foods, we would not have to be concerned later in life about counting calories, eating low glycemic carbohydrates, or making sure we have enough fiber in our diets. However, the problem is that we are conditioned to eating poorly for the most part, and only when health conditions plague us or we become unhappy with our weight do we seek to change those poor habits. Hopefully future generations will learn the importance of good eating habits, and there will be no need to make drastic changes later in life.

Preventing Diabetes With A Low Glycemic Index Diet

Except for juvenile onset diabetes, changes to a healthy eating program can make a difference in whether you develop diabetes later in life. For some people the problem begins during pregnancy with gestational diabetes, and those who develop diabetes during pregnancy have a much better chance of developing the disease later in life. The importance of healthy eating needs to be stressed early in life because the sooner you begin the process of eating healthy, well-balanced meals, the easier it will be to continue doing so.

Diabetes is not a fun disease by any means, and many people don't understand the real complications that it can cause. Even with insulin injections, it's important to eat a diet that is low in sugar content, thus the reason for a low glycemic index diet. Simple carbohydrates such as candy, cakes, and even white bread, starches, white rice, and other high glycemic carbohydrates convert into sugar upon digestion, thus raising the blood sugar level in your bloodstream. Although this may not create a problem when you are young, as you get older, and especially if you continue the practice, you increase your chances of developing Type 2 diabetes. In addition, if someone in your family has it, there is a greater chance that you will develop diabetes as well.

The switch to a low glycemic index doesn't mean that you have to change your entire diet, just the foods that have a high glycemic index such as white breads, potatoes, white rice, bleached flour, and of course, the many sweets such as candies and cakes. What you need to do is substitute high glycemic index for lower glycemic carbohydrates. You can accomplish this by reducing the amount of potatoes you eat, using brown rice instead of white rice, using whole grain breads such as sour dough and whole wheat bread instead of white bread, using whole wheat instead of bleached flour, and choosing cereals that contain oats, barley, bran, and other whole grain products. In addition, reducing the amount of simple carbohydrates such as sweetened cereals, cakes, cookies, candies, and the like and replacing them with fruits and vegetables will also help prevent the onset of Type 2 diabetes. The more ways you find to eat healthier now means the less your chances are of being plagued with the symptoms of diabetes later in life.

The Glycemic Index And Pregnancy

For many people, pregnancy is the beginning of a lifetime of high blood sugar. Those who have never had diabetes yet develop gestational diabetes have a higher than average chance of developing Type 2 diabetes. Of course, if you exert the effort to change your eating habits as soon as you know you're pregnant, or even while you are trying to become pregnant, you may avoid this pitfall. For those who already suffer from diabetes, pregnancy is an added stress factor, and you will need extra care from your doctor during your pregnancy.

More than any other time in your life, it's important during pregnancy to make sure that you eat foods that are healthy for you as well as for the developing baby. This is the best time to get into the habit or eating plenty of fruits and vegetables and substituting high glycemic index carbohydrates for lower glycemic index carbohydrates. It doesn't take much effort to do, and you will find that you have a higher energy level, a very important aspect during pregnancy when a woman tends to feel quite fatigued a good part of the time.

For those who think eating healthier during pregnancy means eliminating your favorite foods, that is not the case at all. For some people it may be a transition, especially those who are not used to eating anything but white bread and rice and pre-sweetened cereals, but it's important for the health of mother and baby to eliminate foods that are high in sugar. In addition to reducing the chances of developing gestational diabetes, switching to a low glycemic index diet during pregnancy can prevent a large weight gain, which can be very difficult to lose after delivery. The consumption of more of the complex carbohydrates that the body is able to convert to energy means you will gain less weight during pregnancy, reduce the possibility of gestational diabetes, increase your energy level, and most importantly, you will learn how to eat a healthy, balanced diet that you can use after the baby is born. Instead of using the excuse that many women do and say that it doesn't matter because you're going to gain weight anyway, use this time to learn new eating habits and become familiar with the carbohydrates that have a lower glycemic index.

The Glycemic Index And Your Health

In some ways, you can link the glycemic index to your health because of its nature and how it affects your overall health. Because we know that too much sugar in the blood can lead to diabetes, it stands to reason that if your diet includes carbohydrates that have a low glycemic index, less sugar will entering the bloodstream, and thus the chances of developing diabetes are reduced. Any time you change your eating habits in order to prevent illness, you are providing the body with the fuel it needs to remain healthy. In addition, carbohydrates with a lower glycemic index include the complex carbohydrates or those that create energy rather than turning into sugar.

The entire purpose of consuming foods that have a low glycemic index is to provide your body with healthy alternatives to the simple carbohydrates that create quick acting energy but cause a meltdown just as quickly. For example, in the middle of the day when you feel tired, you may grab a candy bar to give you a quick burst of energy until the end of the day, but the problem is that you will crash and burn just as quickly when the sugar "high" finishes its job. We do not think of that when we need a quick energy fix, but the fact is that if we take something that is slower-burning energy such as perhaps a slice of whole wheat toast or a bowl or whole grain cereal, it may not give a quick burst of energy, but the energy it gives you will last longer. We think that we need something to keep us from falling asleep, and that sugar-packed product does the job – at the time.

We need to condition ourselves to eating foods that are healthy, and thus preventing the need for quick energy foods. One of the best ways to do this is to get into the habit of eating a healthy breakfast. One of the worst habits that we have is skipping the most important meal of the day. Skipping breakfast is a guaranteed way to lose your energy level before the end of the day, but if you eat a healthy breakfast consisting of whole grains and protein, your energy level will be in its best form for the rest of the day

The Glycemic Index And Heart Disease

Most of us do not think of the foods we eat in terms of heart disease, except the obvious ones such as those high in cholesterol. Failing to recognize the potential for any food we consume to lead to heart disease is a dangerous idea to hold. Although carbohydrates that have a higher glycemic index will not on their own cause heart disease, when they are combined with other risk factors, the potential risk is increased ten fold. The highest potential risk lies in the fact that those who are not eating a healthy diet that includes carbohydrates that have a lower glycemic index are not likely to be eating other foods that are healthy.

The greatest risk factors for heart disease include high cholesterol and high blood sugar (diabetes) both of which can be reduced with a healthy diet and an exercise regiment. A healthy diet begins with one that is low in fat and cholesterol and includes low glycemic index carbohydrates such as whole grains and other complex carbohydrates. The importance of this lies in the fact that simple carbohydrates or those with a high glycemic index value are those that turn to sugar rather than energy and thus have the potential to cause diabetes. The combination of high blood sugar content and high cholesterol make for an unhealthy situation for the heart, and thus the potential for heart disease is increased.

For many people, eating healthy is not something they are prone to do, and unless they grew up in a family where nutrition was stressed, they may not even know that what they are eating is bad for their health. This is especially true of those who do not suffer a weight problem because even though you may feel that because your weight is within normal range, your eating habits are healthy; this is not always the case. Quite often people who are within normal weight range are able to do so because they simply eat less of the foods they consume or they have a very high metabolism that allows them to burn calories quickly. Being within normal weight range does not guarantee that you will not develop diabetes or heart disease, though you may be less at risk than someone who is overweight. To avoid this possibility, follow a diet that is high in low glycemic index carbohydrates and high in whole grains and fruits and vegetables.

The Glycemic Index: Changing Your Eating Habits

When we were children in school, we were taught to eat certain foods to maintain a healthy diet, but unfortunately, as we age, those needs change. Besides, who is going to tell a child to eat whole wheat bread? Sour dough bread? Whole grain cereals? At that age, the important thing was to assure that a child ate three complete meals a day compared to grabbing a candy bar or bag of chips! Children's needs are definitely different from those of an adult, and even adult needs change as we grow older and our bodies go through the changes that are part of the process of aging. As that happens, eating healthy becomes more important, and we learn that some of the foods we are used to eating are not as healthy as we once thought.

Many of us were taught in school nutrition classes that the complex carbohydrates were those of a non-sugar basis such as breads and cereals instead of cakes and candy bars. Although breads and cereals are still healthier than a candy bar, we now know that they still convert to sugar in the bloodstream, and thus we should eat them in moderation. The sad part is that if we had been taught as children that whole grains such as whole wheat bread and oat, barley, and bran cereals were healthier, we would have become used to those products and wouldn't give it a second thought. Because we did not learn that at an early age, we have had to learn it later in life, and thus the transition to a different way of eating is much more difficult. When you have been used to eating high-calorie white bread all of your life, the change to whole wheat or sour dough bread is very difficult. This is especially difficult if you have a family member who blatantly refuses to eat wheat bread, so you have to avoid the temptation to eat white bread because it's in the house.

It's important to learn as early as possible about healthy eating so that the transition to carbohydrates with a low glycemic index is not such a shock for your body. Anytime you change your eating habits, your body has to become used to the transition, and that may take a few weeks before you no longer crave the foods that you used to eat. That doesn't mean you need to give up all of the high glycemic index carbohydrates, but you want to reduce your consumption of them for your body's health.

The Nutritional Value Of Low Glycemic Index Diet Foods

If you're not accustomed to looking at the glycemic index of the carbohydrates you consume, you probably don't understand the importance or have an idea of their nutritional value as it relates to other foods you consume. You don't want to change your eating habits because someone told you that you should do that, but you want to conduct your own research and find out the reason that low glycemic index carbohydrates are better for you.

The most important aspect of the low glycemic index carbohydrates, other than the fact that they are the slow energy producing carbohydrates is that these are the products we often refer to as containing fiber, and as everyone knows, fiber is important for good bowel health. We find fiber in whole grain products, which are one of the major staples of a diet that is rich in low glycemic index carbohydrates. The fiber content in our diets promotes good colon function as well, both of which guarantees that our digestive system works at its best in providing our bodies with the nutrition that it needs.

In addition to the nutrients contained in the foods we consume, the carbohydrates that have a low glycemic index have less sugar, thus the reason they are the slow-energy producers instead of giving a quick pick me up as a candy bar does. The fact that these foods do not automatically convert into sugar also means that the energy will last longer and we will stay fuller for a longer time than with sugar-based products, thus we will need to eat less in order to feel satisfied. For those who have a weight problem or have in the past, that is a definite advantage to consuming these carbohydrates.

For some, the perfect solution may appear to be to give up carbohydrates totally, but that is not nutritionally sound. First, many foods you consume contain carbohydrates, even some things we drink, so you would need to become a label reader. On the other hand, a diet that does not contain carbohydrates is not a healthy one because these are the basis of the energy in your body. To eliminate carbohydrates means you limit the energy within your body, and soon you will be tired and run down and not understand why. Rather than attempting to eliminate all carbohydrates, switch to those with a low glycemic index that are actually good for you.

African Americans And Diabetes

According to the National Diabetes Education Program, there is a current epidemic of diabetes among African Americans. African Americans are one of the largest groups in the population in the United States that are contracting Type II diabetes. In addition, diabetes is also one of the leading causes of death and disability among African Americans in the United States.

There are certain factors that are believed to cause Type II diabetes, which accounts for nearly 95 percent of all cases of the disease. The causes are generally someone with a close relative with the disease, being an African American or being overweight. Other factors include having high blood pressure, high cholesterol and having gestational diabetes while pregnant. It is estimated that about 3.2 million African Americans have Type II diabetes and about one third of them are undiagnosed.

No one is quite sure why African Americans are more likely to get Type II diabetes than any other ethnic group. One thing is certain, however. Poor African Americans are more likely to die from complications of the disease than those in other ethnic groups. This is most likely due to poor health care in certain communities, limited access to drugs that can potentially save their lives and less education. Affluent African Americans have the same chance as other ethnic groups of dying from complications of the disease.

Many people who live in poor communities, in addition to receiving substandard medical care, little education about disease and limited access to lifesaving drugs, also are inundated with fast food restaurants that seem to target certain ethnic groups. Fast foods are usually very high in carbohydrates, fats and offer very little in the way of nutrition. They are inexpensive, however, and many people with little money find this to be the only way they can feed their family on a limited budget. Unfortunately, most of the foods found in fast food restaurants, particularly French fries, are at the top of the Glycemic Index when it comes to foods that should not be consumed by diabetics. French fries are pretty much the staple of any fast food restaurant. They are high in carbohydrates, high in fat and low in protein. But they are filling.

African Americans can prevent acquiring Type II diabetes in many different ways. One way is to take a look at the Glycemic Index and realize which foods are harmful to them and which to avoid. Another way is to start an exercise regime and, if they are overweight, lose some of

Understanding Diabetes and Glycemic Index

those excess pounds. If they are without health care, they should contact their local municipality about screening tests for diabetes. Many clinics and health care facilities offer screening tests for diabetes for those with low income for free. This small step may end up saving the life of someone who is on the verge of getting this potentially life threatening illness.

African Americans can also start saying no to fast foods that, in addition to being precursors for diabetes, are also linked to heart disease, high cholesterol and even cancer. Many fast food restaurants prey on people in low income areas without regard for the health of those individuals. African Americans need to realize that they are experiencing an epidemic of Type II diabetes in their community and do all that they can to stamp it out.

Can A Good Diet Keep Diabetes At Bay

Upon first being diagnosed with diabetes, many patients ask can a good diet keep diabetes at bay. Most doctors will agree that a good diet, low in carbohydrates and sugars can help a person with diabetes avoid many of the complications that often accompany the disease. While a good diet can not necessarily cure the illness, a good diet can keep diabetes at bay.

People who have diabetes have a difficult time processing foods such as sugars and starches. Instead of processing normally through their system, they stay in the system and turn end up increasing the glucose in the bloodstream. When this occurs, it is called glycemia - which is too much sugar in the blood. People with Type I and Type II diabetes both suffer from having too much glucose in the blood. As the glucose does not digest normally, it causes problems with the kidneys, liver, eyesight, heart and blood circulation in general.

Depending upon the stage of their diabetes, a physician will normally prescribe either medication or insulin. Both help the body process the sugars in the blood, to break them down and allow the patient to expel them. However, insulin and medication are no substitute for a healthy diet. Just because a person is taking medication or insulin does not give them carte blanche to consume all of the sugar and carbohydrates they can get their hands on. It is absolutely essential that a person with diabetes not only take medication or insulin as directed, but also adhere to a diabetic diet. This means getting familiar with which foods should be avoided and which foods can be eaten sparingly.

The Glycemic Index was established in 1981 to rate which carbohydrates are the worst for those with diabetes. The carbohydrates that are high on the list, such as white bread, take longer to digest and should be avoided. Carbohydrates that have low scores, such as brown rice, can be eaten in moderation. It is very difficult for anyone to avoid carbohydrates completely, which is why familiarizing oneself with the Glycemic Index is so important in the treatment of diabetes.

In addition to carbohydrates that rate high on the Glycemic Index as well as low, there is also an intermediate group. It may surprise people to know that a chocolate bar is rated in the intermediate group on the Glycemic Index. This does not mean, however, that one should feel free to consume all the chocolate they want. The purpose of the Glycemic Index is to help

Understanding Diabetes and Glycemic Index

individuals establish which foods should definitely be avoided and which foods are okay in moderation.

So, can a good diet keep diabetes at bay. The answer is yes. While it cannot cure a patient of diabetes, a good diet low in foods that have high ratings in the Glycemic Index and high in proteins can help an individual with this condition live a longer, healthier life. Until there is a cure for this potentially life threatening condition, it is important for all people who suffer from diabetes to familiarize themselves with the Glycemic Index so they can better understand how to control their disease.

Diabetes And Sexual Problems

As if people with diabetes do not have enough to worry about, they also have to contend with sexual problems. Diabetes and sexual problems affect both men and women but in different ways. Because your body responds to sexual stimuli through your nerves and high blood glucose levels affect your nervous system, it is understandable that even sexual response is affected by this potentially life threatening condition.

In men, diabetes and sexual problems often focus on erectile dysfunction. It is estimated by the American Diabetes Institute that as many as 85 percent of men with diabetes experience erectile dysfunction. This can cause problems in marriage but, more importantly, can cause severe depression in those who are contending not only with the disease of diabetes, but also what they deem the loss of their self esteem.

Erectile dysfunction can also be a symptom of diabetes. If a man continues to experience this malady, he should discuss this problem with his physician to make sure that he is not suffering from undiagnosed diabetes. Fortunately, there are certain medications and other treatments available to men who experience this common side effect to diabetes. The key to eliminating the problem is for the patient to discuss this with his physician.

Diabetes and sexual problems does not stop at erectile dysfunction, however. Retrograde ejaculation is a more potentially dangerous situation that can happen to men with diabetes. In this condition, the semen can go into the bladder instead of being dispelled out of the penis during ejaculation. A man who is experiencing this side effect of diabetes should seek consultation with a urologist who can help with medication or surgery to correct the problem.

Men are not the only ones affected with sexual problems as a side effect to diabetes. Diabetes and sexual problems also affect women. Because of damage to the nerve cells within the vagina by high levels of blood glucose, dryness can occur that can make intercourse very painful. Many women also report that the nerve damage caused by the hyperglycemia also causes them to lose interest in sex and have no sensations in their genital area. Needless to say, the lack of sexual desire can cause psychological problems for both men and women and may lead to marital difficulties as well.

Understanding Diabetes and Glycemic Index

Many people are embarrassed about speaking to their physician when it comes to problems relating to sexual relations. People with diabetes should be aware of the fact that their condition makes them prone to these side effects and should discuss them with their doctor so they can get treatment. There is a variety of treatment for those experiencing diabetes and sexual problems.

One way to prevent such problems from occurring is to maintain your blood glucose levels by eating a healthy diet, exercising and taking your prescribed medication or insulin. Monitor your blood sugars as instructed by your physician. If you experience any side effects related to your condition, discuss them with your physician. By keeping informed of the disease and the side effects as well as complications, you can empower yourself in managing your illness and lead a happier as well as longer life.

Eye Complications Of Diabetes

Diabetics do not process sugars and starches though their systems like other individuals. These substances stay within their system and enter the blood stream. The high amounts of sugars in their blood, also called glucose, is called glycemia. Glycemia is a condition when someone has an elevated amount of blood glucose. This is often determined by a blood test. People with diabetes have monitors and are supposed to test their blood glucose levels periodically throughout the day to monitor for glycemia.

Glycemia can cause many complications in the body of a person with diabetes. Some of the complications include those with the heart, circulation, blood vessels, kidneys and even eyesight. Because of the high blood glucose levels, a person with diabetes risks having problems with their eyesight. Eye complications of diabetes include those affecting the retina, the vitreous, the lens and the optic nerve.

Eye complications of diabetes take a long time to develop. The first is usually damage to the retina. Tiny blood vessels make up the retina and too much blood glucose cause these vessels to swell. They gradually begin to weaken and the person begins to experience vision problems. For this reason, a person with diabetes should have an eye exam once a year. During the exam, the eyes should be dilated to see if the condition has become worse.

The name for eye complications of diabetes is called diabetic retinopathy. A person with diabetes should rely on a qualified ophthalmologist who is familiar with this condition.

Some of the signs of retina damage from diabetes include blurry vision, flashing lights, dark spots in front of the eyes, pain in the eyes, or pressure and trouble with peripheral vision. If you have been diagnosed with diabetes and are experiencing any of these problems, see your ophthalmologist for a complete eye exam. There are surgeries available that can enable diabetics to be able to regain the sight in their eyes and certain treatments can prevent further damage.

One way a person with diabetes can avoid eye complications of diabetes is to become familiar with the Glycemic Index that rates different foods that should not be included in a diabetic diet.

Understanding Diabetes and Glycemic Index

Exercise is also helpful in diabetic control as is the elimination of alcohol and smoking. Maintaining a desirable weight is crucial to managing your diabetes.

Other eye complications of diabetes include cataracts and glaucoma. While cataracts are relatively easy to cure, glaucoma is a precursor to blindness and needs to be treated. This is why it is so important that someone with diabetes manages their disease with the help of a qualified ophthalmologist.

Many eye complications of diabetes can be avoided if a person with the condition maintains a healthy lifestyle and is compliant in their diabetic treatment. Maintain your weight. Exercise. Eat a proper diet that eliminates carbohydrates and sugars and become familiar with the Glycemic Index. Avoid alcohol and do not smoke. Take prescribed medications as directed by your physician and see your physician at intervals suggested by him or her. Monitor your blood glucose level as often as prescribed. By being compliant in the care of your disease, you can avoid eye complications of diabetes as well as other more life threatening complications of this disease.

Foot Complications Of Diabetes

Whenever we think about people with diabetes, we often think of them as having problems with their feet. This is one of the most common complications of diabetes and diabetes, more than anyone, need to make certain that they address any problems with their feet early on as such problems can result in a life threatening condition.

Foot complications of diabetes are caused by neuropathy. Because the high glucose levels in the blood of a diabetic person affects the central nervous system after a period of time, it also affects nerves in various parts of your body. Most often effected are the nerves in the feet. The furthest from the brain, it is here where people with diabetes who have nerve damage, often do not feel cold or pain or even heat. People with diabetes that is uncontrolled often can injure their feet without feeling it. The injury may result in a blister or wound that will be slow to heal. The blister or wound becomes infected and the foot complications of diabetes begin.

In addition to not having the proper nerve sensations in their feet, people with diabetes often develop very dry feet because the nerves that secrete oil into the feet no longer work. Their feet may peel and crack, which only makes it even more probable for them to get sores and wounds in their feet.

Because high blood glucose levels make it difficult to stave off infection, a diabetic with a sore on their foot must be treated differently than a person without diabetes. The sore may be very slow to heal, if it heals at all. Infection often sets in. This can lead to gangrene and, in some cases, amputation.

Foot complications of diabetes work like this. A person who has diabetes and who has not been keeping their blood glucose level under control gets an injury on their toe. It begins to bleed and crack. Then bandage it, hoping it will heal. It does not heal and soon the wound becomes infected. They go to the doctor who begins to treat the wound with antibiotics. Sometimes this works, sometimes it does not.

When the wound does not heal and the infection begins to spread, gangrene can set in. Gangrene can kill a person, and the doctor knows this. So the person with diabetes has a choice, they can either lose their toe or their life. In most cases, they choose to lose the toe.

Understanding Diabetes and Glycemic Index

In some cases, however, the gangrene has already spread to the foot. Plus, the amputation risks more infection. In many cases, not only does the person lose their toe, but their entire foot. And this can continue until they lose their leg.

This information is not meant to frighten anyone with diabetes. It is only to make a person realize how vital it is for anyone with this condition to be aware of the feet complications of diabetes. No one has to lose a toe or a foot or a leg. They simply need to manage their disease so that they can retain a healthy blood glucose level that will enable them to fight off any infection that may arise from a bump on the foot and stave off neuropathy. By maintaining a healthy glucose level and avoiding glycemia, a person with diabetes can lead a full life. The trick is to follow the rules dictated by the condition.

Avoid foods that are high in starch and sugars. The Glycemic Index is an excellent tool that can inform a diabetic about which foods should be avoided. Maintain your weight and exercise regularly. This will also boost your immune system. Be sure to visit your doctor regularly and monitor your blood glucose level. Keep a record of the levels to present to your doctor so he or she can adjust your insulin or medication if needed. By complying with your physician, you an avoid many of the complications that accompany diabetes.

Diabetes does not have to be a killer. Glycemia is life threatening but can be controlled. If you or a loved one has this condition, see the doctor regularly and follow the plans to manage the disease.

Good Gylcemic Foods

The Glycemic Index was discovered in 1981 and is the basis for many recently popular diets, including the South Beach Diet as well as others. The Glycemic Index determines how long certain carbohydrates take to break down and digest in the system. Those with a high rating, take the longest time to break down and do the most damage to the system of someone with diabetes. The good glycemic foods; that is, those with the lower rates, are more desirable not only for diabetics, but for those who are watching their carbohydrate intake through such diets as the South Beach Diet, they should also be aware of what the good glycemic foods are.

Good glycemic foods tend to absorb slowly into the system, allowing the body to break down the refined sugars and starches so that the body can digest them properly. People with Type I and Type II diabetes have a difficult time digesting carbohydrates, particularly those that are high on the glycemic index, and this lack of proper digestion makes it difficult for the diabetic to expel glucose from their blood,. While most diabetics are wise to avoid most, if not all carbohydrates, as these are what are the most difficult to digest and break down, certain carbohydrates are better than others for diabetics to consume.

Good glycemic foods tend to have a low score on the Glycemic Index that was developed in 1981 at the University of Toronto. Good glycemic foods are still carbohydrates, but make it easier for the diabetic to digest and are much healthier and preferable than those glycemic foods with high ratings on the Glycemic Index. Substitutions are available for foods that rate high on the Glycemic Index and are widely available in supermarkets and other food stores.

Some of the foods that rate low on the Glycemic Index include most fruits and vegetables, Although fruits and vegetables contain sugar, the sugars contained in these good glyceic foods digest into the system at a lower rate and also provide valuable nutrients to the diabetic, or just about everyone. The only vegetable that a diabetic should avoid is a potato, as it has a high glycemic index. Other fruits and vegetables, however, are preferable than white rice, white bread, corn flakes and anything made with white refined sugar or flour.

Other good glycemic foods include wholegrain breads and pastas. If you or a loved one has Type I or Type II diabetes, you should switch to whole grain breads and pastas made from wheat flour. This can be tremendously helpful to anyone who wants to manage their glycemia

Understanding Diabetes and Glycemic Index

as well as anyone who wants to follow such low carb diets. Basmati rice is also considered one of the good glycemic foods.

Often, it is not a matter of eliminating carbohydrates when one is using diet to control their diabetes, but understanding which carbohydrates rate high on the glycemic index. Diabetes is a disease that can be controlled by proper diet, monitoring one's blood sugar and following doctor's orders as far as medication.

How To Use The Glycemic Index

The glycemic index is a rating of carbohydrates that was developed in 1981 by Dr. David J. Jenkins of the University of Toronto. This concept was developed to help people who wanted to rank carbohydrates based upon how they affected the blood glucose levels. Different carbohydrates are absorbed into the system in different manners and all take different times to break down and digest. Carbohydrates that break down and cause rapid digestion tend to leave the most glucose in the blood stream and cause the most damage to a person who is a diabetic. These carbohydrates are given a high rating on the Glycemic Index.

The carbohydrates that are given a high rating on the Glycemic Index include those made with white sugar, white flour, baked potato, French fried potatoes, white break, pastas made with white flour. Even corn flakes are considered bad carbohydrates on the Glycemic Index. This can be valuable information for anyone who has just been diagnosed as a diabetic and wants to discover which foods are more beneficial. While most diabetics will be told to avoid carbs, avoiding carbohydrates all together is not often feasible. For someone who thinks a candy bar is way worse than white bread, the Glycemic Index can be a real eye opener and can be a great way how to use the Glycemic Index for someone who is trying to discover which carbohydrates are safer than others.

Another way on how to use the Glycemic Index is to learn which carbohydrates are better for those who are trying to either watch their carbohydrate intake or who are on a diabetic diet. Some foods, such as fruits and certain vegetables, are low on the glycemic index and take a longer time to absorb into the bloodstream, giving the body the benefit of the nutrients while allowing the body to expel the glucose in a more natural way. One caveat when it comes to fruits and vegetables is that baked potatoes are not considered in the low group in the Glycemic Index.

As a matter of fact, potatoes are one of the highest ranking foods in the Glycemic Index. People consume French fries throughout the world like they are going out of style. Not only are they high in fat and offer little protein, they are also very high in carbohydrates.

Intermediate carbohydrates in the Glycemic Index include foods with a rating from 56 to 69. These include candy bars, some brown rices and croissants. This an be invaluable news to

Understanding Diabetes and Glycemic Index

someone who is learning to develop a diabetic diet but who is unaware of what foods rank high and rank low.

Most people may assume that a piece of white bread is way worse for a person with diabetes than a candy bar, but this is not true. By learning the different ratings and classifications on the Glycemic Index, a person who is watching their carbohydrates as well as their diabetic diet can learn some invaluable lessons and learn how to use the Glycemic Index to their advantage.

Type I and Type II Diabetes

There are two different types of diabetes. Type I and Type II. Type I Diabetes is usually diagnosed in children and very young adults. Type I Diabetes differs from Type II in that a person with Type I Diabetes does not produce insulin at all. Insulin is needed to take sugar from the blood into the cells. Type I diabetes used to be called Juvenile Diabetes as it was diagnosed in children at early ages. The symptoms of Type I and Type II Diabetes are very similar. Frequent urination, frequent thirst, excessive hunger are three of the most common symptoms.

A person with Type I Diabetes must be on insulin for the rest of his or her life. This does not mean that they cannot lead a long, productive life. In fact, people who are diagnosed young in life become accustomed to the treatment and are generally more compliant than those who are diagnosed with Type II diabetes later in life and who tend to ignore many treatment options.

Years ago, a child who was diagnosed with Type I diabetes had to inject himself every day with insulin to remain alive. Today, however, insulin pumps are available that make daily injections a thing of the past. A person with Type I diabetes, as is the case with those with Type II diabetes, has to watch their diet and avoid certain foods high in sugar and starch.

In 1981, the Glycemic Index was developed at the University of Toronto that rated those foods diabetics should avoid on a scale system. Some foods were very high on the scale and took a longer time to process in the system, causing more strain on the kidneys and adverse affects on insulin. Other foods were low on the scale and digested at a slower pace. For years, it was commonly assumed that sweets were the cause of diabetes at that these were the only foods to avoid. With the advent of the Glycemic Index as well as other medical studies, it became apparent that sweets were not the only foods to avoid. As a matter of fact, a baked potato, often seen as a nutritional substance, is actually more harmful than a candy bar.

Carbohydrates are the bane to diabetics. And this is the food group rated on the Glycemic Index. People with Type I and Type II diabetes must limit their intake of carbohydrates. Certain carbohydrates, those rated low on the Glycemic Index, can be taken in smaller quantities. Those on the high scale should be avoided at all cost.

Understanding Diabetes and Glycemic Index

People with Type II diabetes are generally diagnosed later in life. This condition often effects older people and those who are obese. The incidents of Type II diabetes has mirrored incidents of obesity in the United States and most in the medical community agree that there is a clear link to obesity and the development of this disease. People with Type II diabetes do not process enough insulin to break down the glucose in their system and cause their kidneys to work overtime in getting rid of the waste. While some people with Type II diabetes are prescribed insulin, most are started on a regiment of medication.

Physicians generally hope that by taking medication as prescribed, exercising, eating the right foods and monitoring their blood glucose levels, they can avoid the use of insulin. In many cases, patients are very successful at maintaining good blood sugar levels by modifying their diet, exercising and losing weight. Others who are not successful usually end up taking insulin.

As with both Type I and Type II diabetes, there are complications. These complications such as heart disease, nerve damage, kidney disease and skin disorders can be avoided if patients comply with the instructions of their physician, learn about their disease and do all they can to manage it. Diabetes is far from a death sentence. With proper maintenance, those with Type I and Type II diabetes can live long and happy lives.

What Is Hypoglycemia?

Hypoglycemia is a symptom of people with diabetes Type I and Type II. It occurs when people have too little sugar, or glucose, in their blood. While this often is the result of medication from diabetes, hypoglycemia has many different causes and can affect anyone. Those with this disorder present with low blood sugar. This can be temporary and easily fixed by protein or food. In some cases, people who have been fasting can develop low blood sugar. Often, this is quickly cured by protein.

It is a common misconception that someone suffering from hypoglycemia should be given something sweet to alleviate the condition. The truth of the matter is that those suffering from hypoglycemia are usually lacking protein and a food high in protein can alleviate their symptoms. Peanut butter is an excellent choice in helping someone suffering from hypoglycemia.

In some cases, however, hypoglycemia is a disease as it occurs for many different reasons in a person. The best way to define hypoglycemia is to say that it is the opposite of diabetes. While people with diabetes need to avoid sugar as they have an abundance of glucose in their blood, those with hypoglycemia have low glucose levels and need to replenish the sugar or glucose in their blood. In many cases, those with diabetes may develop hypoglycemia as a reaction to insulin or diet. This is different than someone who experiences hypoglycemia on an occasional basis, usually the result of not eating properly.

Symptoms of hypoglycemia include shakiness, anxiety, heart palpitations, sweating, dilated pupils, coldness, feeling of fainting, clamminess. These symptoms are triggered by the loss of glucose that affects the brain If untreated, a person with hypoglycemia can fall into a diabetic coma and even die from the hypoglycemia. If someone is suffering from hypoglycemia, they should be given something to eat rich in protein to avoid falling faint or, in the worst case scenario, falling into a coma.

Other symptoms of hypoglycemia include physical symptoms such as vomiting and abdominal pains as well as hunger. As hypoglycemia continues, neurological symptoms may include difficulty speaking, slurred speech, fatigue, anxiety, lethargy, delirium, headache, stupor, abnormal breathing and finally, coma.

Understanding Diabetes and Glycemic Index

One of the first things that a doctor will do to treat someone with hypoglycemia is to determine the circumstances that caused the disease. A physical examination is necessary and blood samples will usually be taken. Many cases of hypoglycemia are unexplained as no sample is taken from the blood before glucose is given to relieve the symptom.

In many cases, hypoglycemia is nothing to be concerned about. It can simply be the reaction of malnutrition or fasting. Many people experience hypoglycemia without even knowing it. If it continues to be a problem, however, many people will seek medical attention to determine the underlying cause of the illness.

For the most part, hypoglycemia has many common causes and for those who experience the symptoms, testing by a medical professional is necessary to determine the etiology of the cause of hypoglycemia. In a good number of cases, the cause for hypoglycemia is never determined and the situation resolves itself.

Understanding Diabetes and Glycemic Index

This Product Is Brought To You By

DAVID A OSEI

www.ingramcontent.com/pod-product-compliance
Lightning Source LLC
Chambersburg PA
CBHW050507290526
45786CB00006B/2471